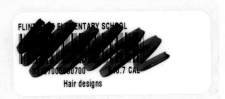

DATE DUE

DISCARDED

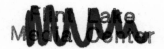

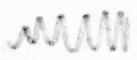

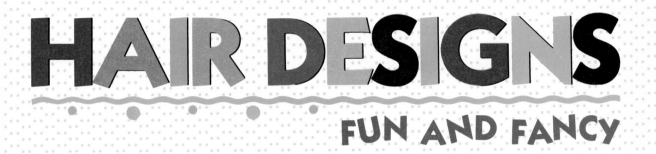

HAIR DESIGNS
FUN AND FANCY

by Margaret Caldwell
Photographs by Marjory Dressler

SCHOLASTIC INC.
NEW YORK TORONTO LONDON AUCKLAND SYDNEY

Credits

Photographer: Marjory Dressler
Fashion Stylist: Lu Rossman
Hair and Makeup by Paola Bacchini for Zoli Illusions
Bow and Ribbon Stylist: Cindy Stern
Assistant Stylists: Barrie Rubenstein and Sue Ogden
Photo Assistant: John Rutledge
Creative Consultant: Michelle Tiberio
Models: Brooke Fontaine, Alexandra Gizela, T.F.Walker: Ford Children
Book design by Dawn Antoniello

ISBN 0-590-47144-9

12 11 10 9 8 7 6 5 4 3 2 1

3 4 5 6 7 8/9

Printed in U.S.A.

08

First Scholastic printing, September 1993

CONTENTS

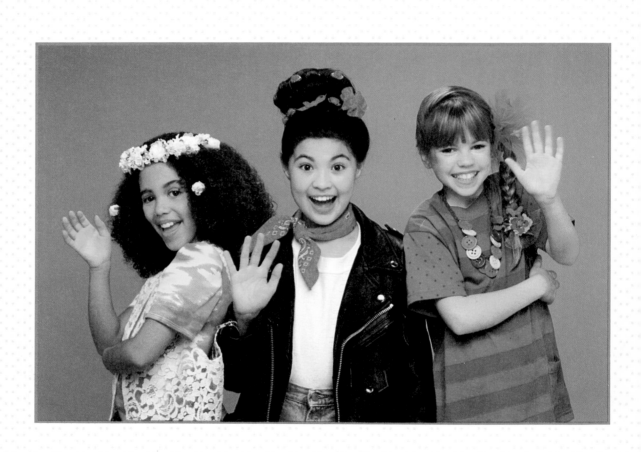

INTRODUCTION

Have some fun with your hair! Gorgeous hair shows you off at your best! Loose and shiny is lovely, or jazz it up with this year's new styles. From ponytails to flips to braids and buns, you can create a new chic style any day of the week. Experiment alone, with a friend, or with your mom.

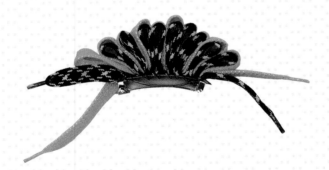

You don't need a stitch of new clothing to stay with the trends. Just stitch up a few barrettes or scrunchies! An old T-shirt or plain sweater looks dressed up with a fun ribbon to add some snap. Test the trends with beads and flowers. Dress yourself up with ribbons and bows!

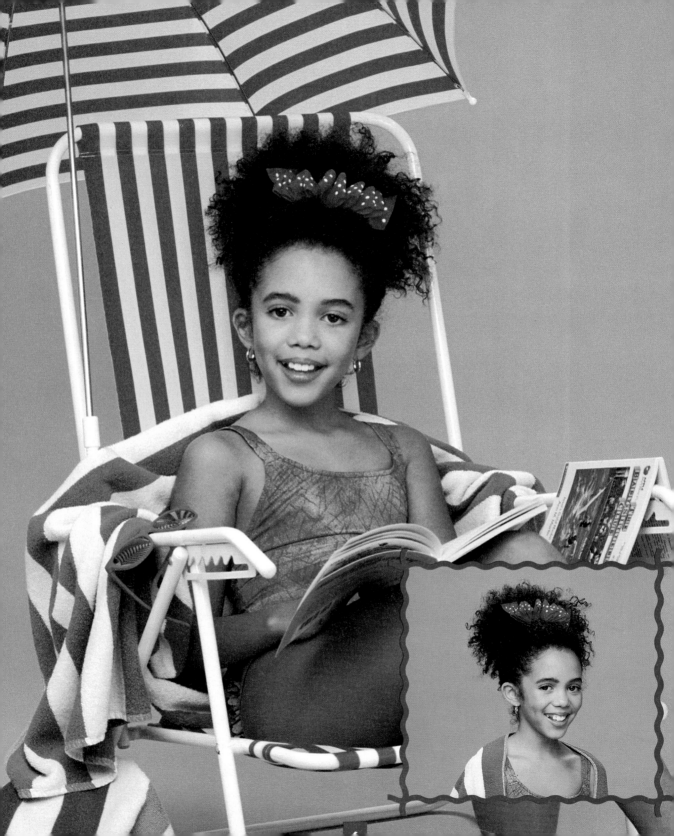

PONYTAILS and TWISTS

A PONYTAIL is clean, sleek, and **easy**! Dress it up with ribbons, or keep it simple for playing sports.

HINT: Make sure your hair is well brushed or combed before you pull it back from your face.

1

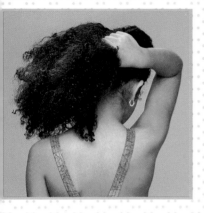

2

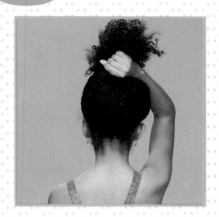

3

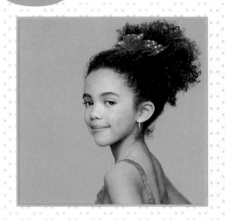

1. Pick the spot where you want your PONYTAIL to flop: in the back, on top, or off to the side.

2. Brush all your hair together at that spot, collecting it with one hand.

3. Secure it with an elastic, ribbons, a scrunchie, or a big barrette.

TRY THESE TRIMS:

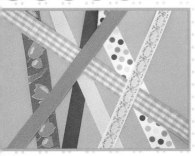

RIBBONS

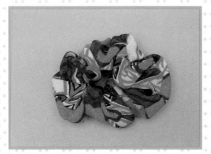

SCRUNCHIES

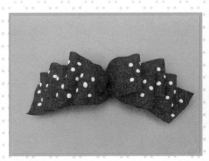

BARRETTES

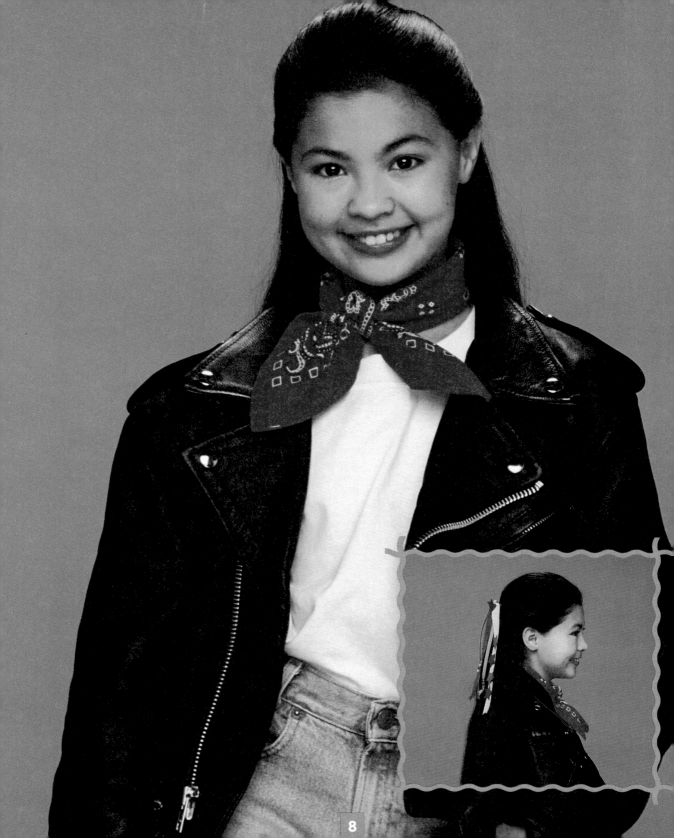

Have the long hair look, but keep it out of your face with a PARTIAL PONYTAIL. This look keeps the hair out of your eyes, and gives you a spot to wear colorful trims!

1

2

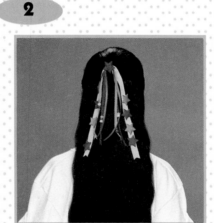

Pick the spot where you want your hair to gather together.
Brush back only one layer of hair from both sides of your face.

Secure it with an elastic or barrette, and Trim It Up!

TRY THESE TRIMS:

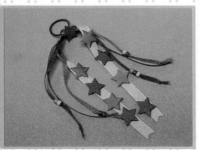

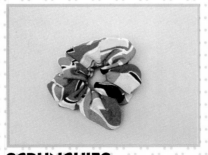

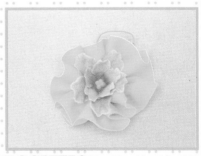

RIBBONS on ELASTICS

SCRUNCHIES

ROSETTES on ELASTICS

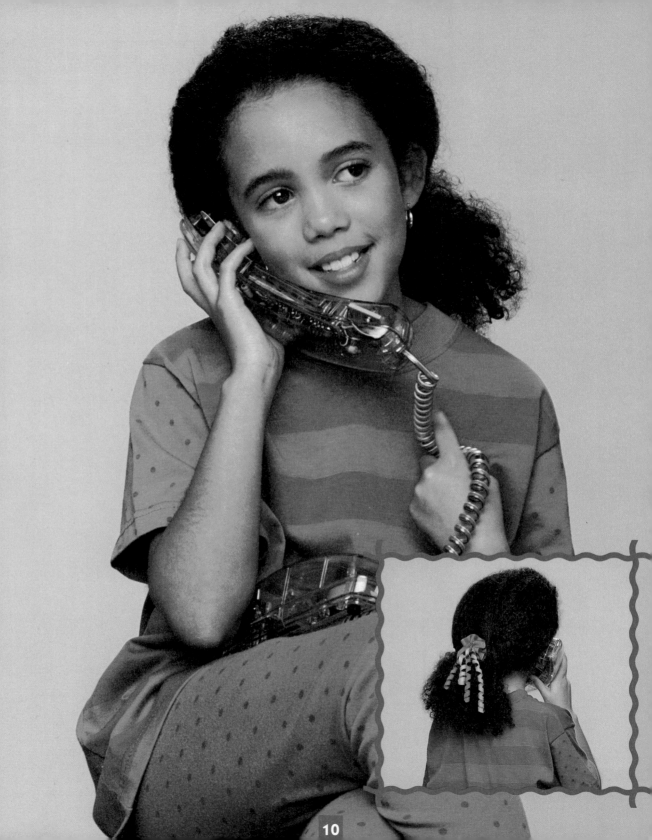

THE PONYTAIL "FLIP"

This FLIP looks complicated, but is a cinch to do! It looks terrific with a FULL or PARTIAL PONYTAIL. It is an easy style made elegant!

HINT: Secure your ponytail loosely to start. If it is too tight, it may hurt to pull your hair through.

1 **2** **3** **4**

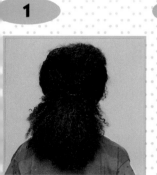 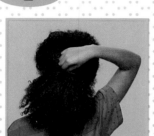 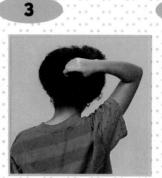 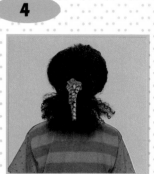

1 Make a PONYTAIL, and secure it loosely with an elastic.

2 Make a "hole" in your hair **above** the elastic, using two fingers on one hand.

3 Reach for the hair **below** the elastic and pull it up through the hole.

4 Flip the PONYTAIL out.

HIDE THE ELASTIC WITH:

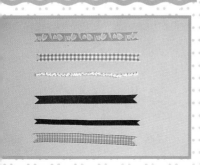 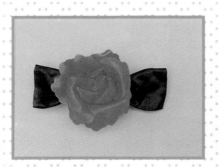 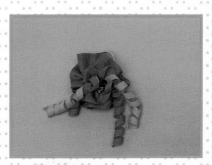

RIBBONS **FLOWERS** **ROSETTE WITH TWIRLIES ON IT**

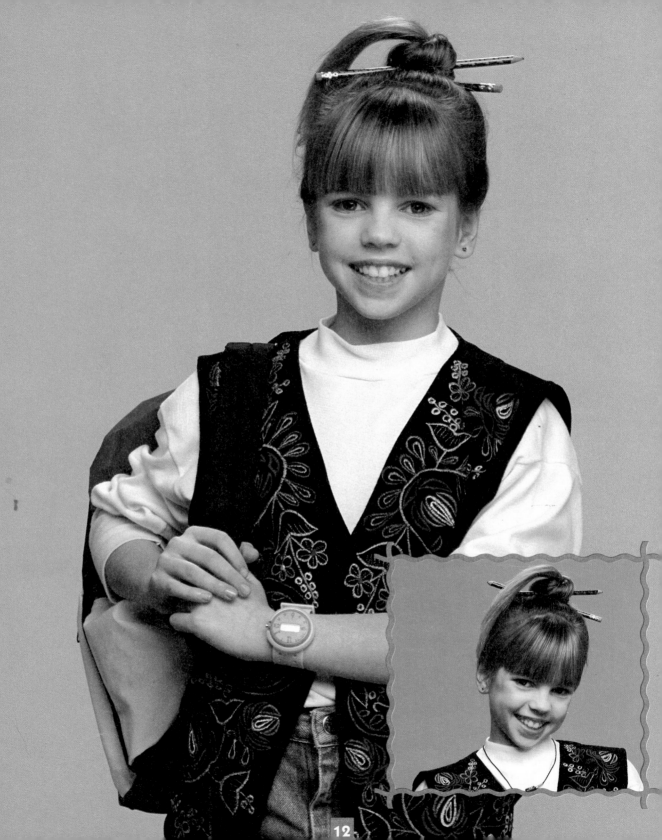

The KNOT is a casual look that works best with longer hair. You can do it in a second in the locker room, stick your pencil through it for decoration, and you are all set for class!

HINT: The KNOT holds itself and is best done when your hair is slightly damp.

1

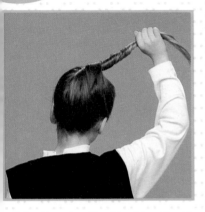

2

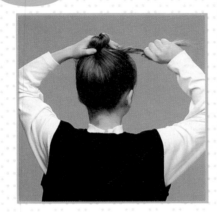

3

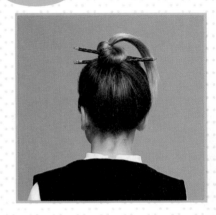

1 Make a PONYTAIL, holding it together with one hand. Now twist the PONYTAIL to the right.

2 Put a finger on the left side of the twist, and coil the twist around your finger, clockwise, to make one full circle. (Use your thumb to hold the hair as you circle around.)

3 Reach through the center of the circle and pull the rest of your PONYTAIL through.

TRIMS: Because this style holds itself together, **less** decoration is best.

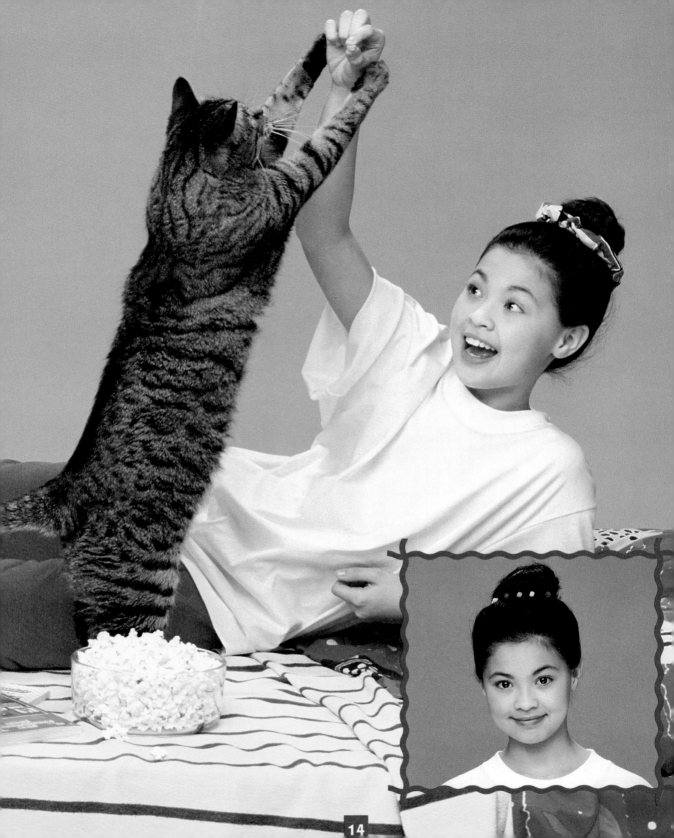

THE PONYTAIL BUN

The BUN is a classic ballerina look, or a great way to show off a new scrunchie. The BUN looks elegant dressed up or left by itself.

HINT: You will need hairpins.

1
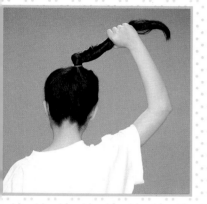

2
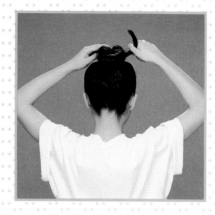

3
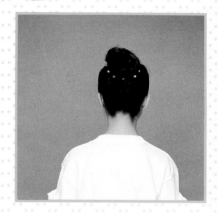

1) Start with a classic PONYTAIL. Secure it with an elastic. Twist the hair to the right, all the way down the tail.

2) Wrap the twisted tail around the elastic, until the full tail is used up.

3) Hide the very end of the tail under the BUN, and secure it with a hairpin. Use several pins to secure the whole BUN.

TRY THESE TRIMS:

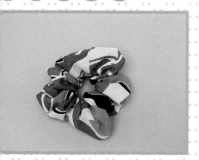

CRUNCHIES

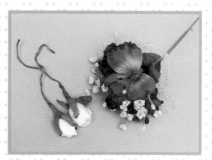

FLOWERS

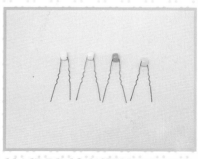

HAIRPINS WITH BEADS

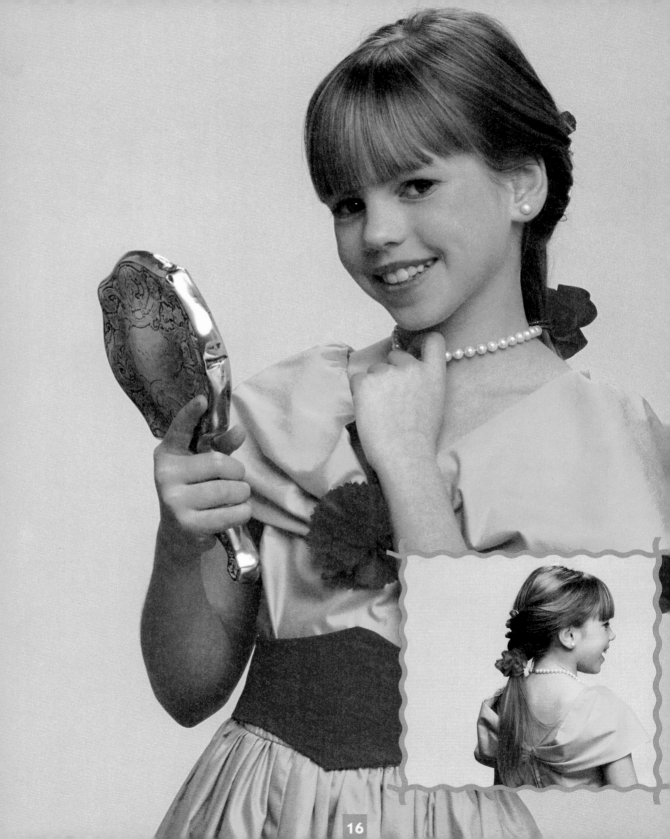

The TWIST is a fancier way of pulling your hair back into a PONYTAIL or a BUN. You can even do it simply to pull a little hair off your face, and secure it with barrettes! It adds a dressy look.

HINT: You'll need a friend to help you!

1	2	3	4

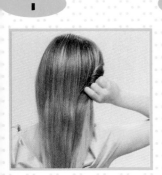 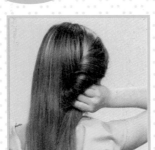 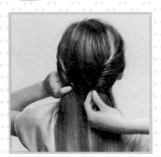 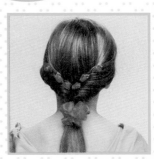

1 Start on one side. Take a front section of hair, pull it back, and twist it.

2 Add a second section of hair to the TWIST, and continue twisting. (You could stop here and secure the TWIST with a barrette, leaving the rest of your hair down.)

3 Continue adding sections until you reach the center back. Now: One person holds the TWIST, while the other twists the other side.

4 Finally, secure the two TWISTS together at the center back.

TRY THESE TRIMS:

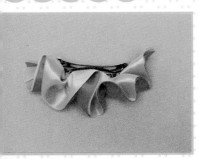  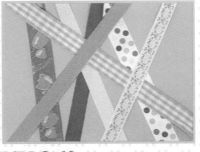 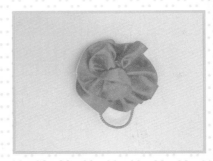

BARRETTES   **RIBBONS**   **ROSETTES**

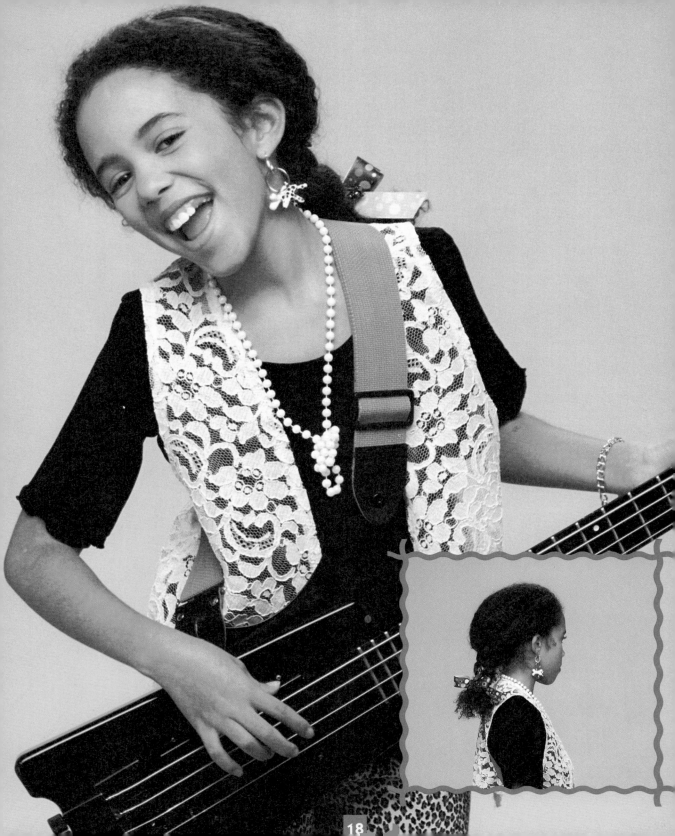

To BRAID means to weave together three strands of hair. The idea is that the three sections make a pattern by switching places in a certain order. You can braid all of your hair or just one section. It will look as classy as can be!

HINT: If you are just beginning to learn how to BRAID, secure your hair in a PONYTAIL first. Practice on a friend!

1   **2**   **3**   **4**

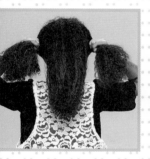 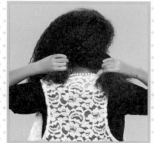 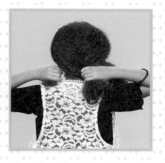 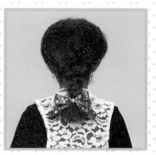

Divide your hair into three equal sections. Hold the side sections, one in each hand.

Cross the right section over the middle section. It now takes the place of the middle section. Pull the "old" middle section over to the right.

Now let's go to the new right section. Cross the left section over the current middle section.

Repeat from step 2, alternating right and left cross-overs until you have reached the BRAID length you like. Secure it with an elastic.

TRY THESE TRIMS:

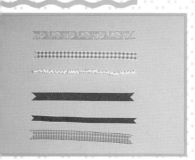

RIBBONS

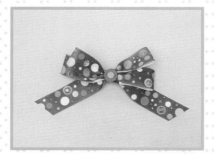

BARRETTES

BEADS on HAIRPINS

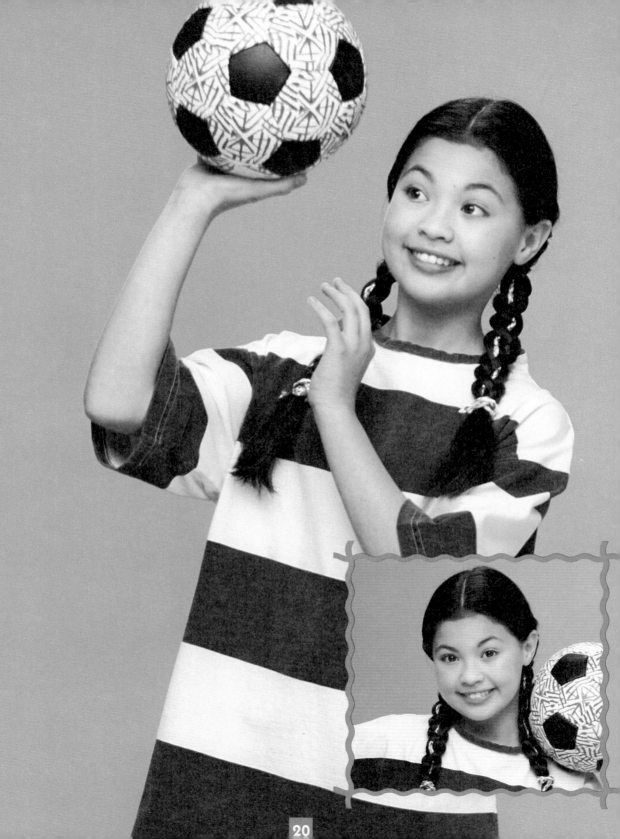

THE **PIGTAIL BRAID**

Pigtails are BRAIDS that are on the sides of your head. You can leave them down straight, or create a lot of different looks shown below.

HINT: Do the braiding behind the ear for a cleaner look.

1	**2**	**3**

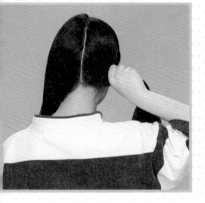 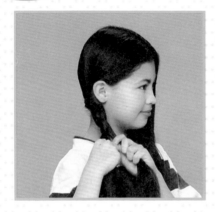 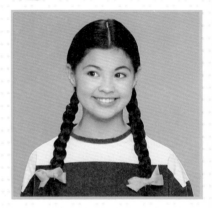

1 Part your hair down the center back and center front, creating two equal sections of hair.

2 Divide the first side into three sections and braid, alternating right and left cross-overs as shown in the CLASSIC BRAID. Secure at the end with an elastic.

3 Repeat the process on the other side. Be sure to start the braiding at the same spot so the two sides are even!

TRY THESE VARIATIONS ON THE PIGTAIL:

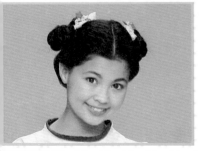 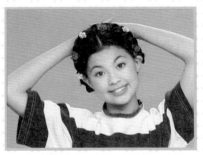 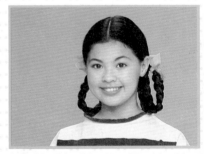

"RUDY"   **"SWISS"**   **"GRETEL"**

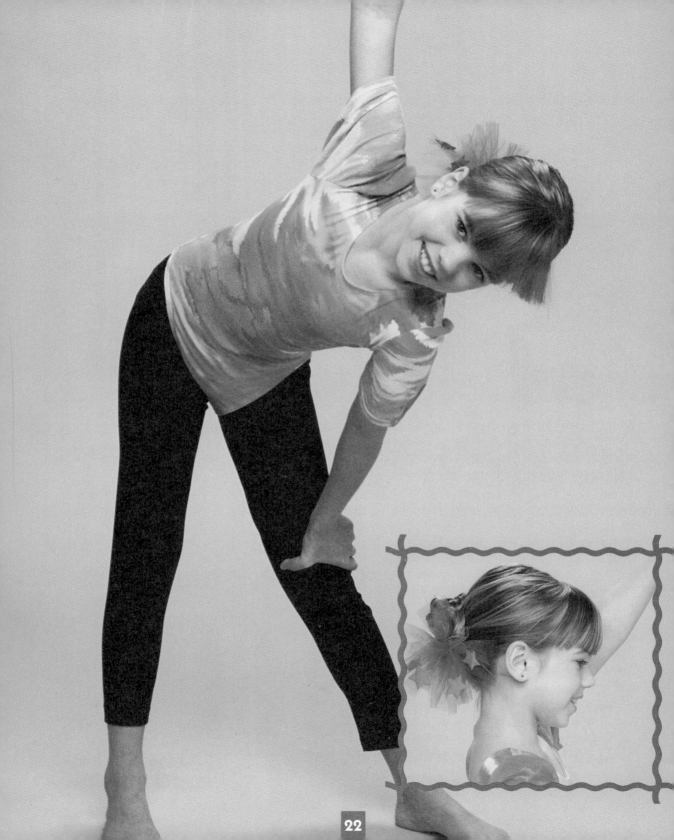

THE **BRAID BUN**

The BRAID BUN is done just like the PONYTAIL BUN, but has a very different look. The BRAID adds texture to the style.

HINT: If your hair falls out of the PONYTAIL BUN, the braid may help give your hair the thickness needed to keep it together. DON'T FORGET THE HAIRPINS!

1 **2** **3**

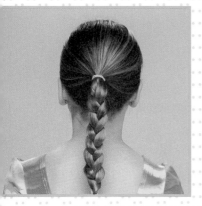 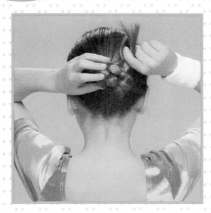 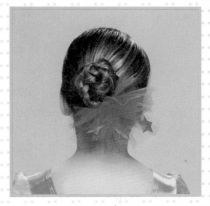

Start with a CLASSIC PONYTAIL, secured with an elastic. BRAID the PONYTAIL down to the end, and secure it with a second elastic.

Wrap the BRAID around the top elastic, until the full tail is used up.

Hide the very end of the BRAID under the BUN and secure it with a hairpin. Use several pins to secure the whole BUN.

TRY THESE TRIMS:

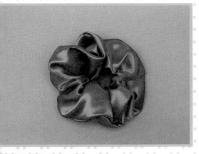 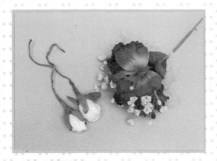 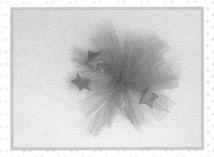

SCRUNCHIES **FLOWERS** **NETTING**

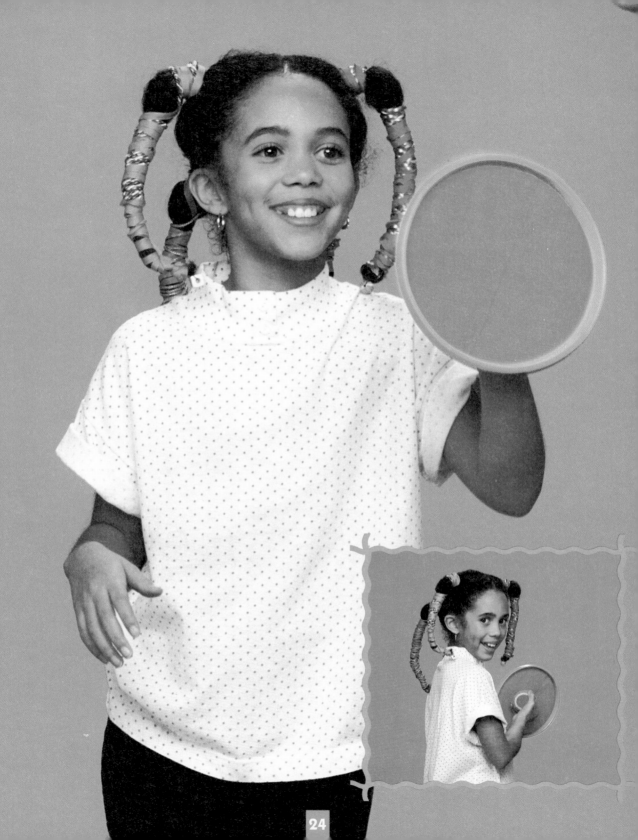

The "OKOTO" PUFF WRAP is a very sophisticated hairstyle from southern Nigeria, a country in western Africa. Lots of girls there, and their older sisters and even their moms, wear this style.

HINT: You can use different colors of cord to make awesome designs. Just be sure to tie the ends of each cord in knots.

WHAT YOU'LL NEED: comb, elastics, scissors, hairpins, and embroidery floss or braided ribbon or cord.

1
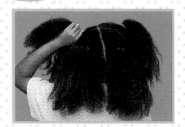

2
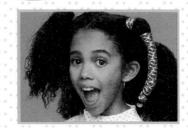

3
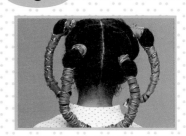

Comb hair out and divide it into sections. Using elastics, secure all but the section you're working on.
HINT: If you have long hair, you can divide it into fewer sections; if you have shorter hair, you'll need more sections.

Take about one yard of cord and twist it around the section several times right at your scalp. Don't wrap the next inch with cord. Now, continue winding the cord around your hair all the way to the end.
HINT: Leaving that inch unwrapped will keep your wraps from sticking straight out from your scalp.

At the end of the braid, twist the loose hairs and tuck them into the wrap with a hairpin.

TRY THESE TRIMS:

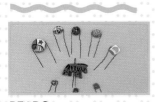

BEADS

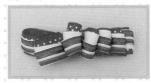

BARRETTES

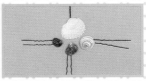

SHELLS

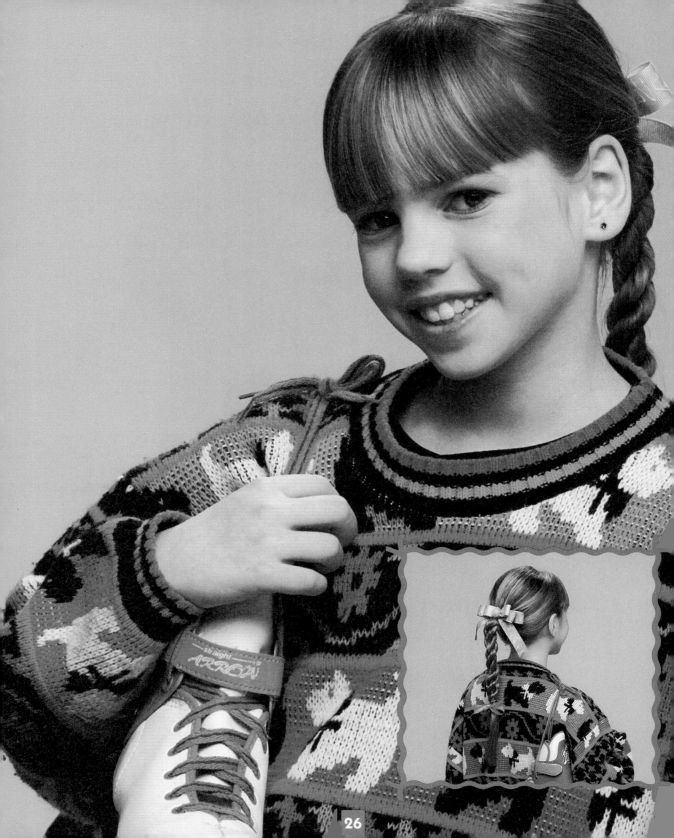

THE **ROPE BRAID**

The ROPE is a really neat style. It looks unusual, and really shows off your hair well!

HINT: This style is easiest to do if your hair is wet.

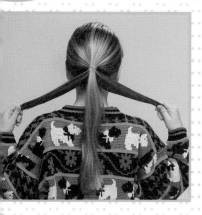   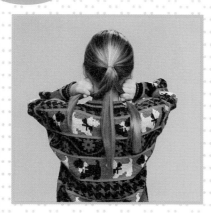   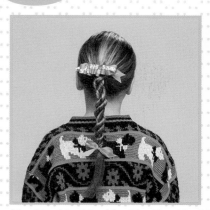

1. Start with a CLASSIC PONYTAIL. Divide the hair into three equal sections.

2. Twist the right section to the right until it's pretty tight. Now cross it over the other two sections.

3. Twist the "new" right section to the right, and cross it over the remaining sections. Continue until you are at the end of the hair. Then fasten your braid with an elastic or a barrette.

TRY THESE TRIMS:

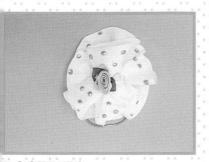   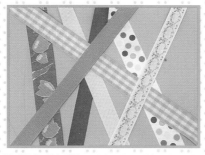   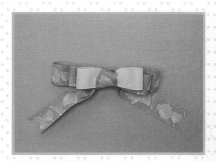

ROSETTES   **RIBBONS**   **BARRETTES**

1.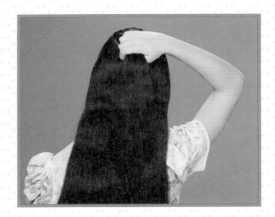

2.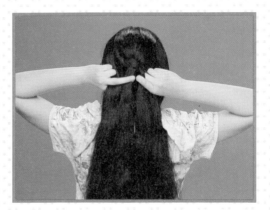

3.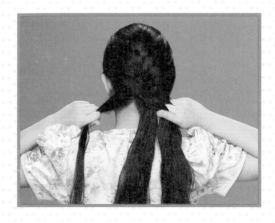

Making a FRENCH STYLE hairdo is not as difficult as it looks. You just need to practice a bit to get the hang of it.

HERE IS THE BASIC IDEA:

Take a small section of your hair and create a style with it (PONYTAIL or CLASSIC BRAID).

Once you have made a mini ponytail, or have done one set of cross-overs for a braid, you ADD A LITTLE MORE HAIR FROM BOTH SIDES OF YOUR HEAD, and REPEAT the style. (Make a slightly larger PONYTAIL, or do one more set of CLASSIC BRAID cross-overs.)

Keep repeating until all your hair is included in the style.

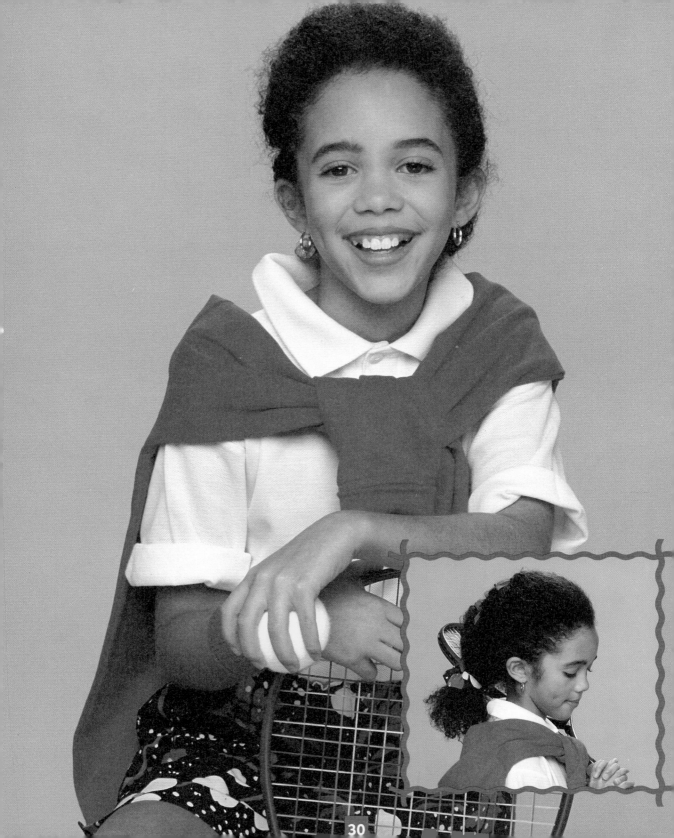

THE **FRENCH PONYTAIL**

The FRENCH PONYTAIL is quite different from the CLASSIC PONYTAIL. Doing any "French style" means you start working with a small section of hair and add as you go, instead of pulling all your hair together at once.

HINT: You will need a supply of elastics, ribbons, or small barrettes.

1

2

3

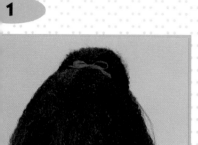

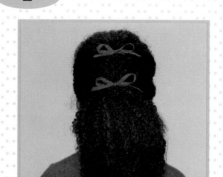

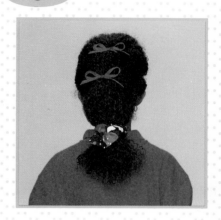

1 Brush together the front sections of your hair, securing them together at the center back.

2 Brush together a second section of hair. Combine it with the first section.

3 Brush together the rest of your hair. Combine all the hair together into one final ponytail.

TRY THESE TRIMS:

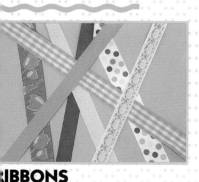

RIBBONS

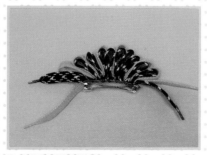

BARRETTES

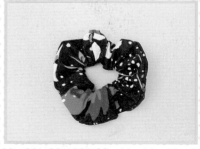

SCRUNCHIES

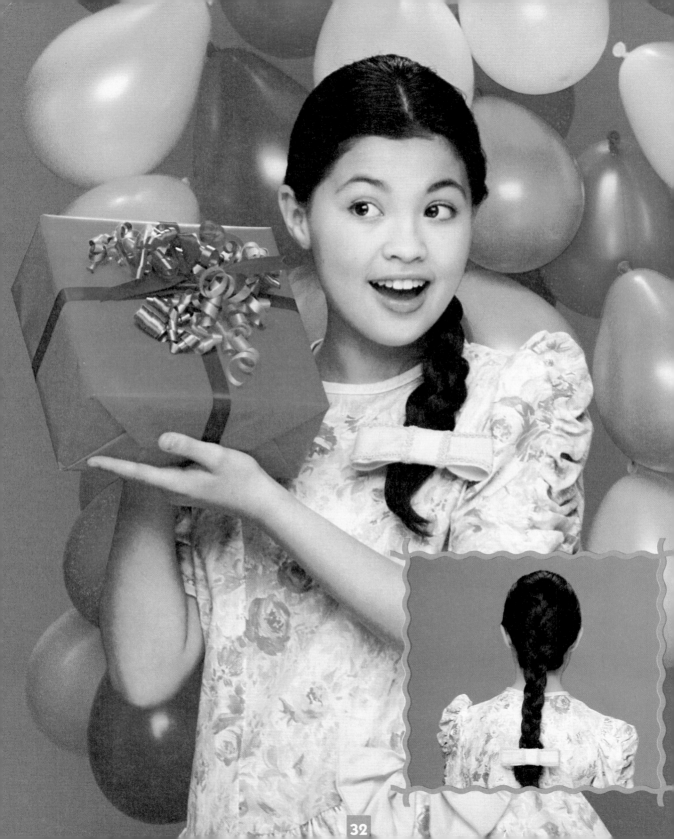

THE FRENCH BRAID

The FRENCH BRAID looks chic with trims or without! It is simply a CLASSIC BRAID, done a little at a time. It is a great style to practice with a friend!

HINT: Keep your hands close to your head as you braid. This will make the braid tighter, and it will hold better.

1

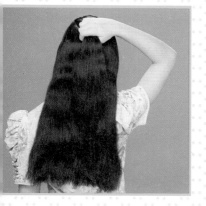

2

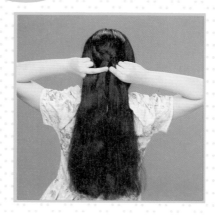

3

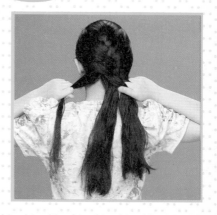

Gather a small section of your hair from the top center of your head. Divide it into three sections, and do one set of cross-overs (right and left) as in the CLASSIC BRAID.

HERE IS THE TRICKY PART: Add a little bit of new hair to each of the side sections, and braid again (one set of cross-overs).

Continue until all your hair is included in the braid. Now you can: Secure it, or do a CLASSIC BRAID for the rest, or tuck the ends under with hairpins.

TRY THESE TRIMS:

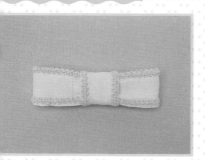

BARRETTES

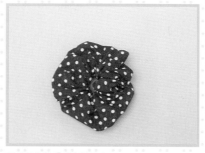

SCRUNCHIES

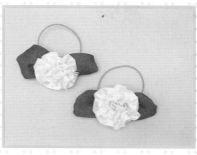

ROSETTES

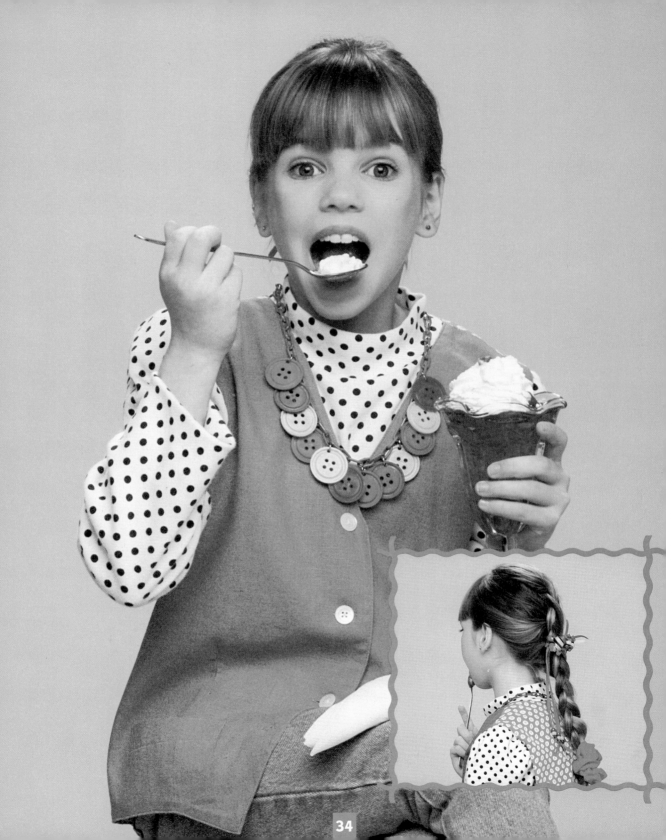

THE "3-D" FRENCH BRAID

The 3-D FRENCH BRAID really makes the braid stand out on your head. It is exactly the same as the FRENCH BRAID, just turned inside-out!

HINT: The trick is crossing the braid sections UNDER the braid, NOT OVER.

1

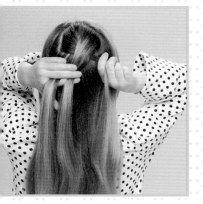

2

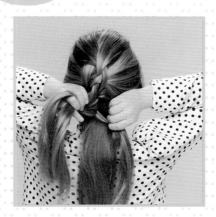

3

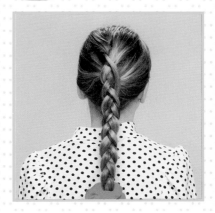

Take a small section of your hair from the top center of your head. Divide it into three sections, and do one set of cross-overs (right and left) as in the CLASSIC BRAID.

HERE IS THE TRICKY PART: Add a little bit of new hair to each of the side sections, and braid again, crossing UNDER not over.

Continue until all your hair is included in the braid. Now you can secure it, or do a CLASSIC BRAID for the rest, or tuck the ends under with hairpins.

TRY THESE TRIMS:

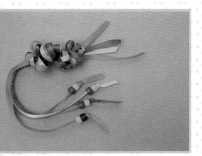

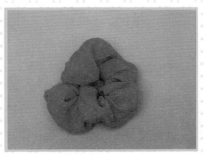

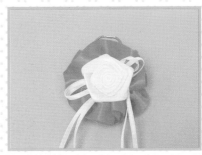

BARRETTES

SCRUNCHIES

ROSETTES

TRY THESE FRENCH BRAIDS

Once you have the idea of doing FRENCH STYLES, you can do all the other hairdos that way. Here are some ideas and hints:

FRENCH PIGTAILS

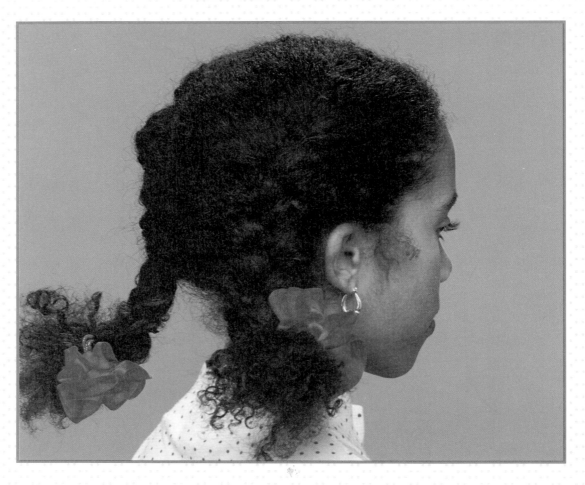

HINTS: Start with a section of hair just in front of the ear running up to the center part. Divide and braid once. Then start adding from top or bottom, moving backward.

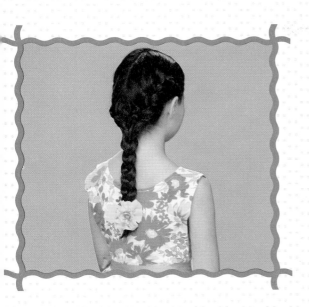

FRENCH CLUSTER BRAID

HINTS: Do FRENCH PIGTAILS until all hair is included. Combine hair from both pig-tails in the back, and do a CLASSIC BRAID.

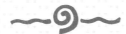

FRENCH TIARA

HINTS: Start with a section of hair combed from one ear across to the other ear. Add only a little bit of hair as you move across the top. A friend needs to do this for you.

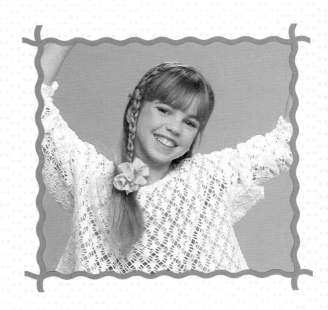

RIBBONS and BOWS

RIBBONS look fun or fancy, depending on the type you buy.

Depending on what you want to create with the ribbons, you may need some supplies.

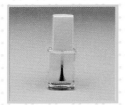

Clear Nail Polish a must!

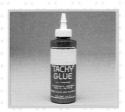

Glue. Almost any type will do, but a fabric "tacky" glue works well.

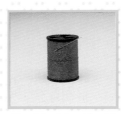

Needle and Thread

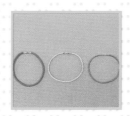

Covered Elastics

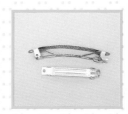

Bare Barrettes

Cut the ends any style, and coat with nail polish to hold the threads.

THE "FAUX" BOW

1.

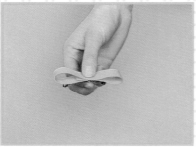

2.

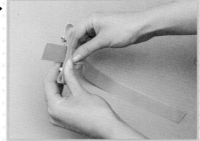

3.

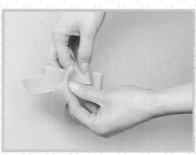

4.

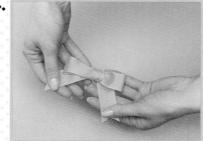

HERE ARE SOME TYPES!

FUN:

1. GROSGRAIN
2. CHECKED RIBBON
3. CRINKLED RIBBON

FANCY:

4. SATIN LOOK

ELEGANT:

5. VELVET
6. FRENCH RIBBON (with wire)

THE CLASSIC BOW

1.
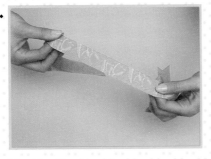

2.
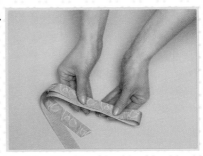

3.
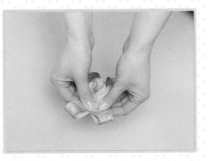

4.
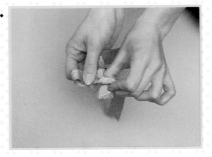

MAKING BARRETTES and ELASTICS

Be creative with the materials you select. Anything can work, with a little effort!!

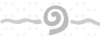

THE TWIST: $\frac{1}{2}$ yard of $1\frac{1}{2}$-inch-wide ribbon or fabric

1. Cut ribbon, and brush ends with nail polish.
2. Sew along one edge, and tie one end.
3. Gather ribbon tightly to desired length, and tie off.
4. Adjust the ribbon in the wave as shown, and attach to barrette/elastic with thread or glue.

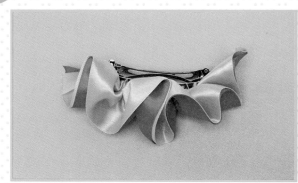

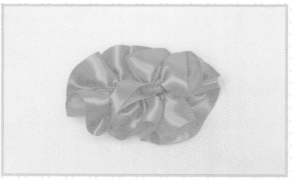

THE SWIRLY: 1 yard of any width ribbon

1. Cut ribbon, and brush ends with nail polish.
2. Sew along one edge, and tie one end.
3. Gather ribbon until twice the length of barrette.
4. Fold gathered ribbon in half, and sew the gathered edges together. Attach to barrette/elastic.

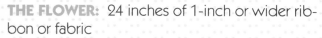

THE FLOWER: 24 inches of 1-inch or wider ribbon or fabric

1. Cut ribbon, and brush ends with nail polish.
2. Sew along one edge, and tie one end.
3. Gather ribbon tightly, and tie off.
4. Coil the ribbon into a circle-like flower. Sew together at the center. Attach one or more to barrette/elastic.

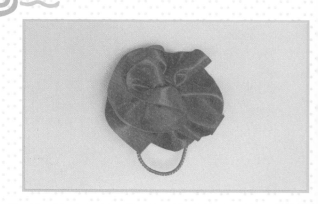

THE SLINKY: 24 inches of any width ribbon

1. Cut ribbon, and brush ends with nail polish.
2. Sew down the middle, and tie one end.
3. Gather ribbon to desired length, and tie off.
4. Attach to barrette by gluing or sewing.

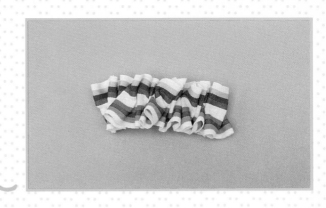

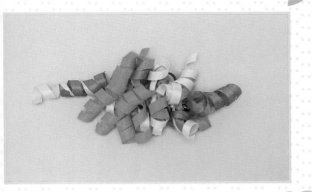

THE FLOPPY: A bunch of 3-inch-long pieces of ribbon, fabric, etc.

1. Cut ribbon, and brush ends with nail polish.
2. Tie ribbon to barrette, covering all or part.

THE NOODLE: 24 inches of any width ribbon (Try shoelaces!). Several ribbons together look great.

1. Cut ribbon, and brush ends with nail polish.
2. Attach thread to one end of barrette.
3. Loop ribbon once, and secure with a double loop of thread.
4. Continue looping to the end of barrette, and tie off thread.

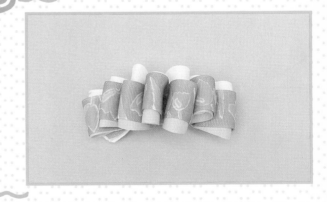

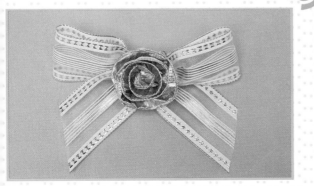

FRENCH RIBBON ROSES: 8 inches of French ribbon

1. Cut ribbon, and brush ends with nail polish.
2. Twist ribbon around your index finger.
3. Sew one edge together with thread.
4. Spread out petals and attach barrette.

BEADS

BEADS can add glitter, color, and flavor to your hair. Try gold beads for a dance, or carved beads for a theme day at school, or lots of colored ones to match an outfit!

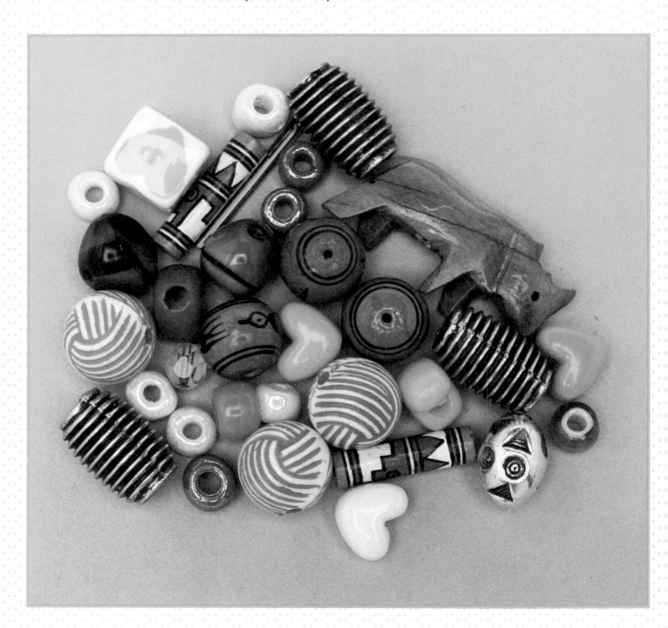

TRY THESE TRICKS:

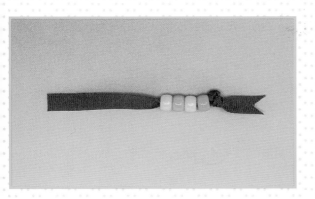

String a $\frac{1}{4}$-inch-wide ribbon with beads, and include it in your braid. (Pin it at the top, or tie it to the elastic.)

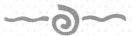

Thread beads into your hair at the ends of braids or around a bun. Hold them in place with hairpins.

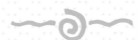

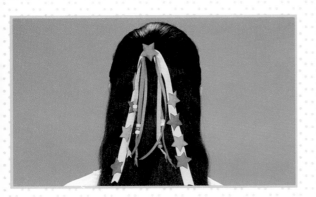

Attach ribbons strung with beads to an elastic or barrettes to add some bangles!

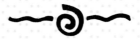

SCRUNCHIES and HEADBANDS

SCRUNCHIES can be headbands, braid-bands, bands around a bun or pigtails. You can make them large or tiny, depending on where you want to wear them.

You make SCRUNCHIES out of FABRIC, so the SKY IS THE LIMIT on patterns, colors, and textures!

Supplies: Fabric cut to 4 inches wide, $\frac{1}{8}$-inch elastic, needle, thread, safety pin.

1. Fold the fabric in half the long way with the right sides together. Sew up the open side.

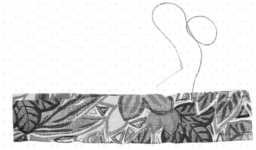

2. To turn the tube right side out, pin a safety pin to one end and push it through the tube.

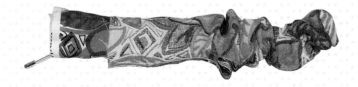

3. Thread the elastic through the tube with the safety pin, gathering the fabric so that the elastic sticks out at both ends.

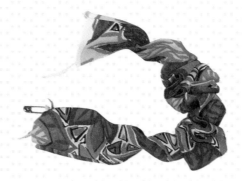

4. Tie the ends of the elastic together.

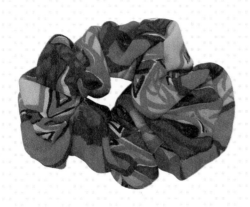

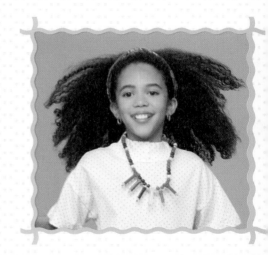

5. Turn the fabric ends under, and sew them together.

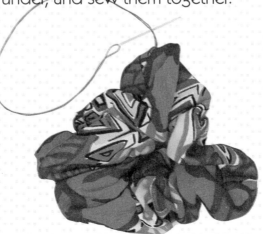

FLOWERS

Real or fake flowers are always *ℛOMANTIC.*

BARRETTES and ELASTICS
Attach flowers to any barrette or elastic with thread or glue. You can even attach a flower to a scrunchie. Don't forget to add leaves!

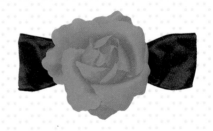

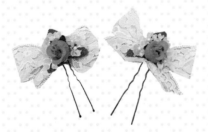

THREADING THEM INTO YOUR HAIR
Thread flowers into your braids by putting the stem through the center cross-over. You can secure the flowers with hairpins.

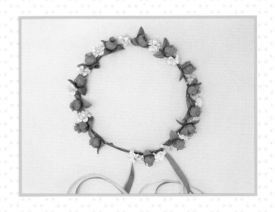

GARLANDS
Make a garland of flowers by attaching flowers to a piece of wire as wide as your head. Your local florist or craft store has special wire and green tape that will make your garland look professional!

LEAVES: A lengh of 1-inch-wide green ribbon.

1. Overlap ends.   **2.** Tie middle tightly.   **3.** Attach rosette or flower.

FANCY HAIR TRIMS

Once you get going, you will soon realize there is **no limit** to what you can use to create fun and fancy hair trims. Here are some more ideas:

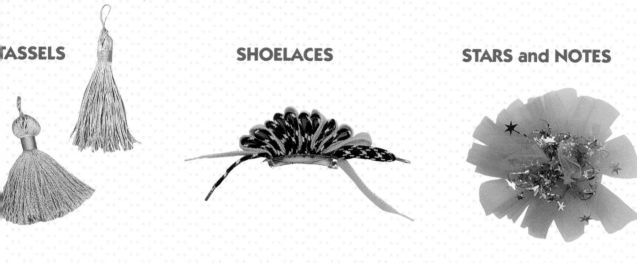

TASSELS

SHOELACES

STARS and NOTES

FANCY UPHOLSTERY "ROPES"

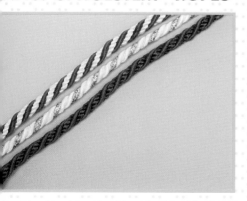

NETTING

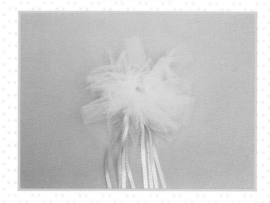

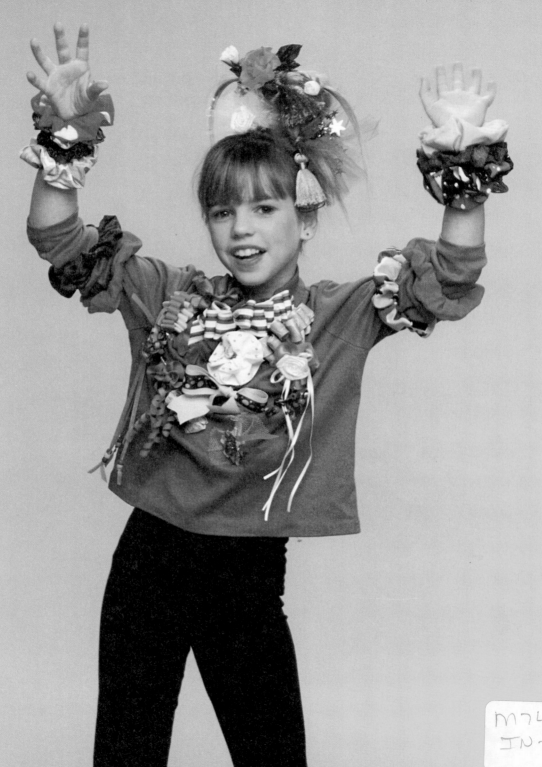